CONTENTS

A BEGINNER'S GUIDE
TO
MULTIPLE SCLEROSIS

How I Put My MS Into Remission Naturally

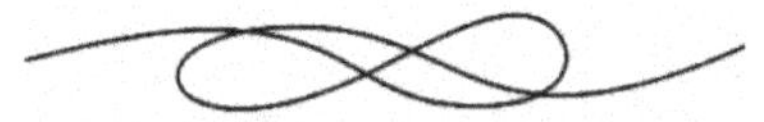

BY: M. SYLVESTER

This book is dedicated to my son and daughter
for always encouraging me to keep going even when
the future did not look so bright.

ACKNOWLEDGMENTS

There would be no book if it wasn't for these people that guided me to remission. First I want to thank Dr. Tressa Pinkleton for helping myself and others when the light gets dim. I want to say a huge thank you to Dr. Cicero Coimbra for his research and persistence to fight this terrible disease and help others. I want to thank John Ottwell for listening to my whining and crying while struggling with your own life.

I want to express my gratitude and appreciation to the following Facebook groups: Coimbra Protocol: North America, Low Dose Naltrexone for chronic illness and infections and Healing Multiple Sclerosis Naturally. These groups were the glimmer of light at the end of the tunnel for me.

Also thank you to my son Cameron Norris for helping me complete this project.

DISCLAIMER

First and foremost, I am not a doctor. I am something even better, an actual person who worked in the medical field and has experienced what you or most people with an autoimmune disorder have experienced. Most of the knowledge and suggestions listed in this book have been from my own research and trial and error. Most people will tell you, 'The best way to heal yourself is to find someone who has done it and copy'. I am one of those people for you as there are many that have put themselves in remission. There will be many different options in this book so that if one doesn't work you can move to the next. Many of you will require multiple actions to get to the point of healing. This is exactly what I did in my search for disease remission, I talked to many different people, I tried different diets, different supplements etc. I measured my success by how I felt, how my energy improved and how my symptoms felt. Healing yourself involves you being your own doctor and many people struggle with this responsibility. But, if you're here reading this book you can, you will and you're already on your way to healing! The first step is believing that it is possible.

Everything listed in this book may work for you, some of the things listed in this book may work for you or none of the things listed in this book may work for you. This is due to everyone having a different metabolic makeup, genetics, the cause of your disorder, the brand of your products and your diligence to sticking with the protocols. So basically, there are no guarantees with anything in this book but it will give you choices, information and hope. Everything in this book can be done with or without being on medications.

This book is for educational purposes only. While the remedies and suggestions in this book have been beneficial to many, still check with your doctor before making any changes to your diet or disease care plan. It's good to make sure that any adjustments that you make won't interfere with any medications or supplements that you already take. As well as affect any other conditions that you may have.

FOREWORD

"The doctor of the future will give no medicine, but will instruct his patients in care of the human frame, in diet, and in the cause and prevention of disease."

– Thomas Edison

Vaccines, chemically processed foods, leaky gut, stress, pregnancy, vitamin and nutritional deficiencies, sleep deprivation, living unauthentically, stress, not enough sleep, toxic products and air, childhood trauma, unforgiveness… Well, you get the point. Or if you don't get the point, it's that sickness and disorder in the body is more than just what we eat. With Multiple Sclerosis the first thing you should know is that it is not caused by one particular thing but by lifestyle. This is so important for people to understand when trying to heal a chronic condition. Many have even started naming these chronic conditions "Lifestyle Diseases" because of how common they are becoming. They were also given this name because a lifestyle change is required to be able to heal. Currently, it is becoming evident that developing an autoimmune disorder requires the perfect storm. The state of unwellness in the body is very much linked to many conditions including our emotional and mental state, what is going on inside the body, along with what we allow around us (friends, family, social media, work). So once one decides to heal, many areas need to be corrected to bring the body back into homeostasis. The only opposition to these statements may be if the sickness is due to genetics.

While there are some doctors that are starting to understand and treat patients with the concept of total body healing, many are still stuck in their traditional ways of treating patients. Then there are also doctors who are knowledgeable of this concept but still try to put patients on strong pharmaceuticals because they receive kickbacks from Big Pharma companies. Kickbacks are monetary payments given to prescribing physicians for prescribing certain drugs to patients. Sickness has become about money in our society and there is no way around it. Autoimmune disorders are becoming more and more common and because of their complicated nature knowing how to help yourself can be crucial to living a longer healthier life. Especially in this day and age where health insurance has become unaffordable for so many.

To be truthful, I believe many autoimmune disorders can be connected to nutritional deficiencies from our foods not containing the same minerals that they did years ago. Furthermore, the chemicals and pesticides that are added have to affect our bodies in some way. Additionally, the stress on most individuals in today's society is high. Stress can definitely affect your health negatively and quickly. Todays society is a lot faster paced than our grandparents was, with suicide and mass shootings on the rise. There's more to it but these are just a couple of the concepts that demonstrate that keeping up good mental and emotional health in this day and time is different from what our grandparents or even parents had to go through.

Autoimmune disorders are very different from having the flu or an earache. There is no cure or any one thing to be given to make them immediately go away. The body is attacking itself and we want it to stop. Many disorders also involve some amount of inflammation as well. Starting as soon as possible on your lifestyle changes when diagnosed with an autoimmune disease can help you be successful with putting your disease in remission before disability starts. The longer you wait to start holistically healing the longer it will take to heal any disability or symptoms. Also, for many, the longer you have one symptom the more it is likely to be permanent. This is not set in stone though. There are many people who have had symptoms for years and are then able to get rid of them or lessen their impact. An important fact to remember is that with MS, everyone is different and one person's outcome doesn't mean that it will be yours.

If you are healthy, this book can help you with preventative steps to keep your health intact. It's always best to not get sick at all, if possible. So keeping our total health in mind can help that.

INTRODUCTION

When I received my diagnosis of Multiple Sclerosis I initially thought my life was over. I was 36 years old, with a new baby, just finishing a degree. How could I, a healthy, active young woman get this disease? I was puzzled. After much research I realized I was the perfect candidate for an autoimmune disorder. Let me explain.

Growing up, at the age of 15 I experienced my first traumatic experience. My father died from lung cancer. This was a very traumatic experience for me as my parents were married, lived in the same home and I watched him die slowly. I remember him coughing violently with blood and mucus coming up. I shaved his head for him during chemotherapy when his hair was falling out. And for some reason we never thought he would die, even though in 1997, this was the typical outcome for a cancer diagnosis. Emotionally, I didnt feel anything for over 10 years and I lost my smile. I acted out and suffered from severe depression and thought about suicide often. My introduction to life had begun. Self-harm became my way of dealing with the emotional pain and I began cutting (self harming to deal with emotional pain) until the age of around 26. I kept this a secret from absolutely everyone and when people would ask me what happened to my arm I would make up lies such as I fell. This is common with people who self harm. From the outside I was a woman with many friends. I kept myself in shape, always had my hair and nails done and was popular where I lived. By the time I was 21, I was a single mother. It took a lot of deception to keep up this public image of being happy at this point. I lived very unauthentically to keep this a secret. By 23, I had already experienced an abusive partner. From there I struggled having random jobs, drug use and random breakdowns from holding in the pain from my father's death. By the age of 30, I was ready to do some major introspectrum. I started prioritizing my health by becoming vegan, working out and praying daily. It seemed I had made it out of the darkness. Another major incident that needs to be looked at in my life is that during this period of putting my life back together, I went back to school to study Radiology . I was required to get vaccines to join the program and to work at the hospital. This is going from not having vaccines in almost 25 years. I had also become an alkaline vegan around this time and was a dedicated follower of the great Dr. Sebi. I made all of my meals from his listed fruits, vegetables and grains. And while I felt great at this time, looking back I'm almost positive that I wasn't getting enough nutrition due to the meals I made. At this time I didn't know much about nutrition and how irresponsibly eating less could put one in a nutrient deficiency or make the current condition even worse. I concentrated on eating less and eating those particular foods. I then became pregnant while I was in school and had my child one year before graduating. About 3 months after childbirth, I began experiencing stomach issues. These were symptoms of extreme bloating and constipation. I eventually got to the point where I couldn't use the bathroom for weeks. I know you may ask, why not seek out a doctor's help? Well, I was so busy with school and the new baby, and I thought many of my symptoms were due to having the baby. I figured it would go away on its own. This is a pretty common situation for most people in today's busy society, ignoring signs from their body or believing they will go away on their own.

A couple of months after the stomach issues I began to experience something else. This was an eye twitch. The first couple of days I didn't think anything of it. Once the eye twitch had been going on for a couple of weeks I began to get concerned. Most internet searches and one of my school instructors suggested that it was stress or not enough water. Both of these things were plausible. I mean, I was under extreme stress daily that I had decided to handle by not sleeping. (I thought I could get more done this way) On top of that I was so aggravated with school, my fiance and just life in general at this point. The eye twitch continued for at least a month until one day it just faded away as well. If I had taken the time to listen to my body, I would have realized that my body was asking for help. I wasn't listening.

Another very alarming symptom that should have made me take action was fatigue. Anyone that has experienced MS fatigue knows that it's not the same as being tired, it's 100x worse. I got to the point where I could barely drive in the afternoons. If you are familiar with Atlanta traffic then you know how bad it can be, especially downtown. It became a daily occurrence that I would have to pull my car over on the side of the road in traffic and sleep. I couldn't make it 15 minutes in my car without feeling like I would fall asleep while driving. Sometimes I did fall asleep at the wheel and to this day I'm thankful that I didn't hurt myself or anyone else. I also tried to start working out around this time and had noticed that I couldn't run. It wasn't that my legs didn't work but it was the fact that I had no energy. I could not bring myself to go faster than a walk and even that I couldn't do for long.

The next symptom couldn't be ignored and made me seek medical help. I was sitting in class one day after working and my vision in one eye just went blurry. Initially, I thought it was my contact lenses. Damn thing must have slid to the side of my eye, I thought. Before I left, I went to the bathroom and looked. My contact was still there but I couldn't see. I called the optician at my eyeglasses store for an urgent appointment. He looked in my eye and said there was nothing that looked strange or abnormal. He told me to go to the optometrist, which I went directly to from there. Once he was finally able to look at my eye he said that it looked like optic neuritis, which is inflammation of the optic nerve. He told me this usually proceeds with some medical issues and he asked if multiple sclerosis ran in my family. I answered no. He then looked at my patient chart and saw that I was paying out of pocket (I had no insurance because I was in school). He was a very sweet man as he said he wasn't going to charge me because he wanted me to go to the hospital where I was going to school and see the optometrist there. They did a lot of low income patients with no insurance. I thanked him, left and hurriedly tried to call the hospital to get an appointment. There were no appointments for six months.

By the time of my next optometrist appointment, the optic neuritis had improved and there were no traces of it. I had googled so much that I was already aware that there was a possibility it could be MS (multiple sclerosis). When it was finally time for my scheduled appointment they told me that many times optic neuritis preceded a multiple sclerosis diagnosis. But, they said, it could just be a one time incident. This is known as CIS (Clinically Isolated Syndrome), I found out later. Basically, they said, the only way to know was to wait to see if I had any more symptoms. I left thinking about what was said, Multiple Sclerosis? How was this possible? When I started school, a year and a half before, I was an alkaline vegan that only ate from Dr. Sebi's list of foods. I worked out at least four times a week before school and was still trying to work out with my busy schedule. My eating had gone left since being in school and working but, a chronic disease? All of these thoughts bombarded my brain but as time passed things went back to normal and nothing else happened. My eyesight slowly came back and life seemingly went back to normal and I didnt think about MS anymore.

Graduation was coming soon and I was excited to be done with this hectic part of my life. Studying and testing day and night was hard with the baby but I was doing the best I could and looking back on it I was doing a pretty good job. Then one morning I woke up and my leg felt numb from the knee down. I was scared but I felt like I had to go to school. Testing was today and my instructor said no one could miss it. I remember walking from the parking lot, to the bus, to the school and it was hard to walk. I was scared. What was going on? Was I becoming disabled? Would people notice? These are all of the things that ran across my mind as I struggled that morning. I was late to school but I had to be there. Looking back, stress was a sure sign of triggering an autoimmune disorder for myself. Stress was abundant at this time in my life. Also dealing with a struggling relationship and a newborn. I had stress at home, nevermind school. I arrived at class and tried to look normal walking. No one noticed to the best of my knowledge. When I was able, I contacted the optometrist again to schedule an appointment. They had told me to contact them again if I had any new symptoms and this was definitely a new symptom. It would be at least four to six weeks before they would be able to see me. This is the day I knew something was majorly wrong. I was scared at this point. MS came to mind again. Was I not going to be able to walk? Was this the start of needing a wheelchair? I hadn't told my family yet as I didn't want to scare them. As women, we take on so much and I had a job(s) to do. Symptoms began multiplying fast after this day. It was like my body and mind were falling apart. I remember sitting in the car one of those days when I had to pull over for a nap and talking to my son, I couldn't remember words. Word recall and brain fog had begun. I would forget what I said the minute before. It was hard to talk. He was the first person I eventually told my big secret too. I cried. What was going to become of me? Would I need someone to take care of me? Would I be able to take care of my son and my baby? Would my fiance even want to be with me anymore? It was stressful in itself to start thinking of myself with this serious illness. My hands then went numb. It was hard to hold a pencil or pen and it definitely was no longer possible to pretend that I didn't have anything wrong with me. I continued to go to school and try to do everything as normally as possible. Continuing my normal schedule helped me keep my mind off the fact that I was deteriorating physically and mentally. I thought, would I even be able to complete my school test since I was finding it so hard to talk, think and remember? During class, I started feeling dumb. Things I would normally know I couldn't figure out. The instructor would embarrass me by asking did I study. I was so ready to be out of this situation so I could focus on my health.

Graduation came and we celebrated. At this point I was getting used to my lower leg being numb and my hands were improving slightly. The night of graduation my baby got sick. We took her to the hospital with a fever and they said they didn't see anything. The next day the fever came back. I felt like something was really wrong. We went to the hospital with her late at night and she ended up having to be put on a breathing machine. They rushed us upstairs to the ICU and told us that if we had come later she could have possibly died. The stress was on 100% once again. Was I going to lose my daughter? I cried and cried. I couldn't eat, I couldn't talk, I couldn't sleep. More stress. They let me hold her because her heart rate would go down when she was being held. We ended up finding out that she had a rare staph infection in the back of her throat. They would give her antibiotics that would work and then the infection would come back. They came to the conclusion that surgery would be best to remove the infection. The surgery was successful. We could finally go home after a month of being in the hospital. One interesting thing I found out was that my daughter's vitamin d levels were at 4 when she came into the hospital. This meant her Vitamin D was almost nonexistent. I had found out earlier my vitamin d levels were low as well. Optimal levels would have been around 50 for her. Was this why her and I were going through these health scares? This information stuck with me and helped me with putting my MS in remission.

Arriving home, my condition seemed to decline even more. I couldn't carry my baby downstairs because I would feel like I was going to fall. I would feel hopeless and depressed most of the days, as school was over and I now was in the role of a stay at home mom. I joined many facebook groups on MS and one in particular had a mentor program for women that have just been diagnosed. I talked daily to an older woman that would listen to me cry, hear my fears and answer my questions. She would reassure me this isn't the end, it was just a tougher path. She said you at least have 10 years left until you will need a wheelchair. This did not help soothe my mind in the least bit. It actually made me more scared. I went to the hospital through the ER and I remember waiting for so long. Why? Because none of my symptoms were visible. As with most autoimmune disorders, no one can see what we're going through.The intake nurse asked why I was there and I answered, " I think I have Multiple Sclerosis". She looked me up and down and said, "Nah, you don't have that. No way". I said, "I hope you're right". I received a lumbar puncture and then a head mri. They gave me IV steroids to calm down my symptoms. I started feeling better after the steroids. My hand numbness went away, I was energetic and my thoughts seemed clearer. They also gave me my official Multiple Sclerosis diagnosis. "Try to eat healthier", the student doctor said to me, giving me a pity smile. They sent me home with a steroid taper (prednisone pills to help you gradually come down from the high dose steroids they gave me in the hospital), a neurologist appointment to receive meds and a large bill. The following days I started to have a moon face (puffy, bloated face from steroids) and a headache. I couldn't lift my head off of the pillow. I was taking the taper daily but I decided to not take it one day due to how bad I was feeling. The headache disappeared! I started researching everywhere I could about MS. I also started talking online to many people dealing with MS. There I found many people who were healing themselves and many with stories of their experiences with the disease.

When it was time for my neuro appointment I felt a lot less hopeless. I actually had already decided on a couple of drugs I was interested in taking. I was excited to talk to the neuro. I was sure she would be interested in my story about how all of the stress, low vitamin d etc. had contributed to me getting this MS diagnosis. But, to my surprise she told me eating, stress and my low vitamin levels had nothing to do with me getting MS. I told her the med that I decided to take and she told me that it wasn't strong enough. She said even though I recovered from my previous symptoms with the steroids, my case of MS seemed like one of the stronger cases. She said I needed to get on meds as soon as possible. I asked her if I could possibly wait to think about it and she told me most people who wait regretted it. She also added that there was a possibility that I wouldn't be able to walk in a year. She recommended one of the strongest meds, Tysabari, and said most of her patients did well with it. I signed the paperwork to get on the meds. It seemed like I had no choice. It would take an IV infusion monthly and I would come back in a week or so for blood testing. This scared the hell out of me. I was petrified and back to feeling hopeless and depressed. Meanwhile, the entire time I was at home, the drug company was sending me gifts. The following week I went to get my blood testing done. They had a pharmaceutical representative talk to me about all of the side effects that could possibly happen. Cancer, PML, weakened immune system...I began thinking this over. Cancer... that is as serious or worse than MS itself! PML... that is definitely worse than MS. If I got PML(a deadly brain infection) I would just die, there was no cure or treatment! I left the office contemplating what I would do. I couldn't commit to taking the meds knowing this information. It just didn't feel right for me. I went home and started researching holistic routines for MS. I joined more FB groups and talked to people who had put themselves in remission. I started the Wahls protocol, Coimbra protocol, changed my water and let go of as many stresses as possible. Later on one of my FB groups had a post that shared a website that tells you how much your doctor gets paid from different pharmaceutical companies. I found my neurologist's name on the site. The drug company that makes the med that she said I needed to take was paying her over $300,000 a year! Now it made sense as to why she thought I needed to start taking the meds immediately. This was my first introduction to the world of big pharma and how the hospitals and doctors all play their part in it. I began to question everything. One thing I realized is that my success with dealing with my disease would be all up to me. I had to be proactive in searching, learning and trying things on myself. I had to be willing to tell a doctor to order a test or order it on my own. This book is to give those of you searching for something to go by, a guide to help you achieve remission. No matter if you choose to take meds or not, many of the things I am about to tell you will help with improving your health or at the least maintaining it.You will also be more knowledgeable about Multiple Sclerosis and the alternative ways people are choosing to heal. Hopefully, it will also give you ideas to investigate for yourself.

WHAT IS MULTIPLE SCLEROSIS

Multiple Sclerosis is a disease of the central nervous system affecting the brain, spinal cord and the optic nerves[1]. All of these make up our central nervous system[1]. People from all walks of life can get MS. All races, ages, socioeconomic levels, vegans, carnivores basically anyone! There were many misconceptions years ago that African-Americans or Asians couldn't get MS or that MS was extremely rare. We are now finding out that these statements are not true. There are some risk factors that have been identified for MS such as age (usually occurs between 20-40), sex (women are 2-3x more likely to have MS with it being rrms), family history (higher risk if your parents or sibling have it), certain infections (Epstein-Barr), race (white people of Northern-European descent are at highest risk), climate (MS is more common in temperate climates such as Canada, Northern US, New Zealand, southeast Australia and Europe), vitamin d levels (having low levels of vitamin d and low exposure to sunlight), genes (a gene on chromosome 6p21), having other autoimmune diseases (thyroid disease, pernicious anemia, psoriasis, type 1 diabetes, inflammatory bowel disease) and smoking (smokers who experience an initial symptom are likely to experience another confirming rrms)[3]. While research has shown that these are common factors in people with MS, some people diagnosed have none of these risk factors.

Exactly what causes MS is unknown. What is known is that something happens in the body which makes the immune system start attacking itself. The immune system starts attacking the myelin sheath which surrounds our nerves causing the signals from our brain, traveling down the nerves, to be interrupted. This causes issues between the brain's messages getting to the rest of our body[1]. Depending on where the damaged myelin is and how severe it is, determines which part of the body is affected and how strong one's symptoms will be in MS[1]. Some people who have the most severe MS can not walk while others who have mild forms of the disease live a fairly normal life. This shows how greatly unpredictable MS is and how its affects range from person to person. Neurologists use the EDSS (Expanded Disability Status Scale) to measure how much someone is affected by their MS and also to monitor disability over time[6]. The EDSS has a scale of 1-10, with the lower score being less disability and the higher scores meaning greater disability[6].

Getting A Diagnosis

If you have been diagnosed with MS or are awaiting a diagnosis, what was your first symptom? Most people who end up with an MS diagnosis have eye disturbances as their first sign that something is wrong. My first symptom was my vision going out in one eye and then coming back and then going out in the other eye and coming back. Next it went out in one eye and I couldn't see for weeks, it slowly came back though. I've also had my near sighted vision or my far sighted vision leave for hours and slowly come back. Double vision, blurry vision, loss of vision, pain with eye movements etc these are the most common first symptoms of MS. Not everyone starts off with vision problems though, many have numbness and tingling, loss of sensation, weakness in the arms or legs, bladder issues, fatigue, loss of balance, vertigo, cognitive changes, sexual dysfunction and more. Having one or two of these symptoms alone does not diagnose you as having MS. But having symptoms, along with positive additional testing could lead you to the confirmation of the disorder.

Getting an official Multiple Sclerosis diagnosis is not easy to receive from doctors for many people. There are many people who have been living with the symptoms of MS for years and still do not have an official MS diagnosis. One thing about MS is that its symptoms mimic many diseases. Many doctors are aware of this so they like to test thoroughly before giving a diagnosis. Additionally, the symptoms of MS vary so greatly from individual to individual that there is no exact template to describe the course it will take in each patient.

Most neurologists or doctors use at the bare minimum an MRI and a spinal tap to determine if a patient has MS. Additional blood is also drawn as well to look for inflammatory signs. An MRI is typically the first test done to determine if someone has MS. MRI stands for magnetic resonance imaging and is usually not painful. This test is done with a machine that you will lay down inside of. It will produce images of the brain that can show the lesions that were formed from inflammation. Most doctors will encourage their patients to do an IV which will put a contrast called gadolinium into the body to increase the visibility of the lesions in the brain. Gadolinium is a rare earth metal that aligns with an MRIs magnetic field but it is also toxic[2]. There has been much debate in the MS community on if the contrast is necessary or not and some patients refuse it. Another test that is typically done is called a spinal tap or a lumbar puncture. This test can be painful as it is a needle inserted into the spine to take out spinal fluid for testing. Most doctors will have the area punctured numbed to lessen the pain though. Once the fluid is captured it is sent to be tested. If a specific group of proteins called oligoclonal bands is found in the fluid, then that demonstrates there is an abnormal immune response going on in the central nervous system[1]. This result alone does not necessarily mean that the patient has MS, but that there is inflammation in the body[1]. But this result coupled with MRIs and symptoms can then lead to a diagnosis for most.

Possible Causes of MS

While multiple sclerosis is one of the most common debilitating autoimmune diseases, its causes are said to be unknown. It's hard to understand how a disorder that affects so many, to this day has no cure. I mean with all of the technology and advances that we have in our society it would seem that a condition such as this would have a cure. But, if we look at how the medical and hospital systems are set up we can understand that everything in the medical system is for profit. If there was a cure, that would of course stop many non-profits, doctors and pharmaceutical companies from making money. While there are drugs that can help get rid of your symptoms, MS in the medical community is said to not have a cure. Many, including myself, have surmised that MS has many different causes depending on the person. Most likely MS comes from a condition the body gets in from an overload of many stresses, toxicity, or nutritional deficiencies. And most people including yourself may find that a precursor to your MS symptoms may have included a very stressful situation or even digestive system issues. Most people have multiple circumstances to get them here. If MS or other types of autoimmune disorders are not genetic (meaning your mother, father, aunt, uncle or grandparent has it) then it is a great possibility that the cause of your MS is something else.

While there are numerous assumptions as to why people get diagnosed with MS, there are some common themes that seem to recur. Interestingly enough, there have been many theories as to why people get diagnosed with MS.

There is one theory that says that MS is related to the dairy protein leaking out of the gut and then producing an immune response in the body. To counter this, care is taken to not eat any dairy products. Another assumption says that MS is caused by saturated fats, and that high levels of saturated fats affect the body negatively. To counteract that, a very low level of fat or a type of Keto diet is eaten. Others stay away from certain oils making claims that this is why the body is attacking itself. Still, another states the disease is a blood vessel issue. This belief says that MS symptoms are caused by blocked or narrowing arteries in the body and that widening the veins will help lessen the severity of MS symptoms. There is a surgery for this called CCSVI that many people have done successfully. Still, the MS medical community insists that this belief has nothing to do with the cause of the disease. There are many other people that believe that MS is a parasite infestation. This belief is centered in the thought that parasites are in the intestines or in the blood. They usually try to treat this issue by parasite cleanses and taking out sugar. An alternative assumption contends that it is an issue of absorption in the gut. Because many sufferers of MS have to take large doses of vitamins to feel better, some surmise that since the colon is where absorption of nutrients is, their disease is caused by this issue. Additionally, it has been documented that a great deal of people have gut issues such as constipation, bloating, IBS etc. along with or before having symptoms of MS.

Stress is also a precursor to many people having MS symptoms. Decreasing stress and anxiety has also been related to a decrease in relapses.

The 4 Types of Multiple Sclerosis

The International Advisory Committee on Clinical Trials of MS in 1996 has categorized MS into 4 different types based on how the disease progresses or does not progress in the body[1]. The types are listed as clinically isolated syndrome, relapsing-remitting MS, secondary progressive MS and primary progressive MS[1]. Currently, there is a international committee organized by the National MS Society and the European Committee for Treatment and Research in Multiple Sclerosis that has proposed that MS be classified in a new way[1]. The new way would describe MS as a continuous disease that produces damage to the nervous system and describe how well each individuals body can repair itself or compensate for the damage[1]. I think this shows advancement in the MS community as everyone's body reacts differently to the disease depending on other lifestyle factors. We've seen this proven in people such as Matt Embry, who was diagnosed with MS in 1995[5]. He has been living symptom free for almost 24 years which he accredits to his diet, exercise, CCSVI and lifestyle[5]. One main thing about this disease, is to not get trapped into a negative mindset. If you're in a negative mindset about your diagnosis, you may not try new protocols or stick as closely to your diet because you believe it doesn't make a difference. But having a positive outlook, believing that you can do this because others have done this and educating yourself from those that are living successfully with the disease, makes all of the difference. Truly, if you're reading this book looking for information on how to heal yourself, you're already showing your willingness to win at putting this condition in remission.

Clinically Isolated Syndrome is given as a diagnosis when an individual has neurologic symptoms caused by inflammation and demyelination and the symptoms last for 24 hours[1]. It is also given as a diagnosis when healed lesions in the brain are seen or inflammation is seen in another part of the brain other than the part which should be causing the symptoms[1]. Having this condition does not mean that you will be diagnosed with MS but there is a high probability that the person will have another episode. Another difference in those with CIS is that many times there are no brain lesions. Brain lesions are of course a main characteristic of MS (which is why they get MRIs if they suspect it), so if these are absent there is less of a chance of a MS diagnosis.

Relapsing-Remitting MS (RRMS) is one of the most common types of Multiple Sclerosis. It is said that initially 80-85% of MS patients are diagnosed with RRMS[4]. One of the traits of RRMS is that it relapses (periods of symptom worsening) followed by periods of partial or complete recovery, or remission[1]. Relapses can also be called exacerbations or attacks in the MS community but it usually all refers to the same events. RRMS may progress to secondary progressive MS, but it doesn't in everyone.

Secondary-Progressive MS (SPMS) is what occurs once relapsing remitting MS progresses. Secondary progressive is diagnosed when neurologic functions or symptoms become progressively worse or disability accumulates over time[1]. It is said that this usually happens at a period of 10 years, but once again this is not set in stone and does not have to be your story. A person with SPMS may still have periods of remission, but they will be few and farther apart than a person with RRMS.

Primary- Progressive MS (PPMS) is a type of MS where disability and progression starts from the beginning of the disease course. Approximately 10% of new MS diagnoses are categorized as PPMS[4]. PPMS also takes a minimum of 12 months to diagnose compared to RRMS which can be diagnosed faster[1]. Also a diagnosis of PPMS is required to have 2 of the following: a positive spinal tap, lesions on the spinal cord or lesions on the brain[1]. These are not required for a diagnosis of RRMS. This type of MS also doesn't usually respond to meds. Currently there is only one med for use against PPMS.

HEALTHY EATING MAKES A HUGE DIFFERENCE

As most people know, diet makes a difference with your autoimmune disorder. There are so many diets to try that it does become a little overwhelming. I bet you're wondering what to try first. You'll speak to others who say this worked or didn't work for them. But that doesn't mean that their outcome will be yours. You see, everyone's diet choices should be based on what your body needs. It is a proven fact that vitamin or mineral deficiencies can cause some of the same symptoms that are common from many autoimmune disorders. The diets that are shown may be adjusted to fit your requirements. Getting food allergy tests done can be beneficial as well. Most people kickstart their diet by taking out dairy, gluten, sugar and processed foods. Some other common intolerances are tomatoes, mushrooms, chicken, shellfish, pineapple,strawberries, potatoes, lentils, black beans, corn, avocado, rice, peanuts and buckwheat. But ultimately, you will have to try a couple of these diets and see how you feel after implementing them. This could take months because it would be best to try each for at least 3 weeks.

While there are many diets that could possibly help you, I've included the ones that people with MS have said that helped them. My favorite diets are the diets created by doctors who were diagnosed with MS or doctors that have family members with MS. And actually, these diets are the most popular in the MS community as well. And even though I use the word diets, I would consider these to be lifestyle changes that you would need to make.

Elimination Diet

The elimination diet is a good way to start off. If you are concerned that some of the foods you have been eating are harmful to you this would be beneficial. Also many times, we are not aware that foods are harmful to us until we stop eating them and try them again. To do the elimination diet start off by taking whichever food you are concerned about out of your diet for a minimum of 2 weeks. Add the food back in and see if any of your symptoms get worse or stay the same. If your symptoms get worse then you know you should take the food out entirely.

Green Smoothie Diet

The Green Smoothie diet has been very popular with those that have very severe symptoms. It involves eliminating everything out of your diet and just putting in fruits and vegetables. Many people have said they were able to resolve some symptoms, pain or numbness from eating this way. To start the Green Smoothie Diet, you would replace each of your meals with a green smoothie. These green smoothies would contain at least 1 green leafy vegetable such as kale, spinach or chard combined with other vegetables or fruits. The base of your smoothie should be water, tea or coconut water. If you became hungry while following this plan you could eat fruit, nuts or have a salad. Try to continue this diet for at least 2 weeks but most people who it works for notice changes in 1 week. If you have success with this diet you could possibly have a deficiency in vitamins K, A, C or E. One issue with this diet is it may be hard for some to stay consistent with. In choosing a diet you want to make sure that it is something that makes you feel better and can work with your lifestyle.

Raw Food Diet

Many people have had great success with eliminating symptoms with a raw food diet. This diet is just like the name says…raw. So nothing cooked, baked or fried. Learning how to prepare food so that it is tasty is most of the battle. Eating salads with all raw ingredients and no meat, spiraling cucumber and adding tomatoes and using nuts to make sauces is also in the diet. Because nothing is cooked this diet is full of nutrients. When our food is cooked it takes out much of the nutritional value so eating in this manner can greatly help if you believe you have a severe nutritional deficiency. Most of us with an autoimmune disorder do.

Veganism

There are many people who live by veganism with and without an autoimmune disorder. But, there are also people who I have seen in a relapse (a period of worsening symptoms or symptoms coming back) eating this way and it has helped improve their symptoms. Veganism involves eating no meat. Sometimes people eat fish and call themselves a vegan but, that's not a vegan. Vegans eat no meat (or fish) or any other animal products. Animal products include eggs, milk, cheese or anything made from an animal. The best vegan diets are those with lots of veggies and fruits. There are many 'vegan' foods that are also processed. Just because these foods are vegan doesn't mean that they are healthy. This is where the term 'junk food vegan' came from. Also, when you are vegan you should try to eat a wide variety of foods to avoid being nutrition deficient. This will just worsen your condition.

Blood Type Diet

The Blood Type Diet is a fairly new concept which involves eating based on you guessed it…blood type. The Blood Type Diet was developed by a naturopathic physician named Peter D'Adamo. This diet recommends different foods and exercises based on blood type. According to this logic Type O blood is primarily 'the hunter' and they should consume lean protein and veggies and avoid dairy and grains. Type A blood is considered the agrarian and should consume mostly plant based meals but some fish would be allowed. Type B blood is considered 'the nomad'. This blood type is said to be best with chicken, turkey, salmon, dairy and leafy greens. They should avoid gluten and nightshades. Lastly, is type AB blood which is named 'the enigma'. People with this type of blood are said to do best eating dairy, tofu, fish, lamb, grains, fruit, and vegetables. Many people live by the Blood Type diet but others think it has no basis. Because many people have benefited from changing their diet in this way I feel it is definitely worth looking into.

The Wahls Protocol

The Wahls Protocol was introduced to the public in 2014 and is for all chronic autoimmune issues but was personally used by the author, Terry Wahls MD, to put her Multiple Sclerosis in remission. Dr. Wahls talks about how she was in a reclining wheelchair diagnosed with progressive MS before changing her diet and other things in her life. Personally, I love reading books from authors who have helped put themselves in remission. They are usually very passionate about what they are writing about. Another interesting fact I noticed is that when most doctors are diagnosed with these conditions they do everything that they can to heal themselves naturally. That speaks volumes with the knowledge that they have. Her book basically involves eating in a paleo nature leaning towards a keto. She has 3 tiers to the diet as well going from least restrictive to the most restrictive. I had success with this diet but difficulty with keeping it up. She suggests that all meat be organic and grass fed. Organ meats and seaweed are also included. Moving up in the tiers, fruit gets pretty restrictive and you're restricted to eating berries. Fats are allowed in the diet and she lists which ones you can have.

Her book also talks about exercise, stress and has recipes and meal plans. So many people believe in this diet that she has grown a following on social media and has branched out to having others teach her protocol around the world.

Swank Diet

The Swank Diet is named after Dr. Roy Laver Swank and originated in the 1940s when Dr. Swank was studying MS. Under his thought process, he suspects that fats have an impact on the amount of symptoms and flares a person may have. He suggested having less than 20g of saturated fat a day and for the first year no red meats. The Swank Diet includes eating lots of fruits and vegetables and only 3 whole eggs a week. Egg whites were fine because they contained no saturated fats. There were also supplements added including cod liver oil, as this has high levels of vitamin A, vitamin D and omega 3 fatty acids which all have been proven to help reduce inflammation. By the 1950s his diet was being used in medical settings across the country with results concluding that disease progression was slowed down and patients were less likely to die. This was at a time when those diagnosed with MS were basically doomed. Amazingly, there was a 34yr long study done following the patients who stuck with the Swank Diet and many of the people who stuck with the diet seemed to have improvements, less disease progression or better health compared to those that didn't.

OMS

OMS stands for Overcoming Multiple Sclerosis and is a diet based on what Professor George Jelinek did to put his MS in remission. It builds on the previous diet, Swank, and has a couple of changes. Like no saturated fats or cod liver oil. Instead Jelinek recommends a whole food, plant based diet with flaxseed supplementation, seafood, meditation and exercise. His belief is that fats and oils can lead to the development and progression of MS and other autoimmune diseases. He really has an amazing and hopeful story I feel, as his mother had MS and he watched her deteriorate and later die while growing up. Later on in life he started having MS symptoms and was eventually diagnosed as well. As of right now Jelinek is in good health and leads conferences around the world. Currently, this is the diet that I follow with a couple of additions because it is simple. I love eating fruits and vegetables and I like seafood. Remember, One thing you have to think about when choosing a diet for yourself, is what you can be the most consistent with.

Best Bet

The Best Bet Diet was created by Dr. Ashton Embry when his son Matt Embry was diagnosed with MS in 1995. Dr. Embry wanted to help his son the best way that he could so he started studying MS and came up with the premise that leaky gut may be the cause of MS (amongst many disorders). Many researchers may not agree with this but Dr. Embry has a good thesis behind his belief. He believes that tiny pieces of food leaking out of the digestive tract and entering the bloodstream through leaky gut are causing the body to produce an immune response. The immune response is the body attacking itself because it confuses the protein in the food pieces with the protein in the myelin. This diet is also whole food, plantbased with chicken and fish added. But the plan eliminates dairy, gluten, beans, peanuts and sugar. Supplements include vitamin d, calcium, magnesium and omega 3 amongst other things. Another idea included is exercise. The plan urges that exercise be done at least 20 min a day. One thing I love about the Embry family is they are really in this to help people heal naturally and you can tell by the work they do with others. They give out free Best Bet Diet books and cookbooks. I've also seen Matt Embry help patients with severe MS get connected with resources that can help them. Also, in 2017 Matt Embry produced a very popular documentary called Living Proof which investigates the financial gain and politics of Multiple Sclerosis. I suggest that you watch it if you are truly interested in how disease and big pharma work together.

Carnivore

Many people will look at me crazy when I talk about how a carnivore diet has helped many put their autoimmune disease in remission. A Carnivore diet is usually followed by one only eating meat, fish and dairy products like eggs. There are some variations where some will also eat non-starchy vegetables, organic honey and berries. Carnivore is based on the idea that we should eat like our ancestors and that carbohydrates are causing many conditions that are around now. I have personally talked to someone who has put their disease in remission by eating only organ meat. I know you're probably wondering how this could be possible but it actually makes perfect sense if someone's MS is from being nutrient deficient. See, organ meat is very nutrient dense containing B- vitamins, folate, magnesium, iron, selenium, zinc, vitamin d, vitamin A and more! Carnivore is currently being used to heal not only MS but other autoimmune disorders such as Arthritis, Psoriasis, Inflammatory Bowel Disease, Crohn's Disease, PCOS and more. In my diet I added organ meat at least 2 times a week. Organ meat is very nutrient dense and contains all of the amino acids that our bodies need. It also contains B- Vitamins, iron, choline, copper, folate, vitamin A and CoQ10. CoQ10 is a powerful antioxidant that can help prevent cardiovascular disease and cancer.

In conclusion, the most important thing is to find what makes your symptoms improve and be consistent with whatever you choose. That way you'll be able to see the negative or positive results. Also, think of some of the symptoms that you experienced prior to being diagnosed. Did you have digestive system issues like myself? Did you have tingling and numbness for years before? Keep track of your symptoms and if they get better or worse with your dietary changes. These notes can help you look into what diet may help your symptoms more.

GUT HEALTH

Gut health is becoming such a big topic these days and for good reason. Scientists are now linking many diseases and disorders to problems with the gut. Leaky Gut, IBS, Sibo, Crohns, Celiac disease, constipation, bloating and more are now being connected to complicated conditions such as Multiple Sclerosis, Lymes, Lupus, Rheumatoid Arthritis and others. I bet you're wondering, "How can something from the gut affect our nerve cells in the brain?" Well one presumption that I think is highly likely is that some people naturally don't have a strong gut lining or that gut issues cause the lining of the colon to have holes or to be thin. Food particles then leak out of the digestive system into the bloodstream and go through the blood - brain barrier causing inflammation in the brain (MS Hope). Another assumption that has been made is that saturated fats and processed oils are irritating the digestive system and causing issues in the gut (Overcoming Multiple Sclerosis). Despite which hypothesis you may believe both are linked to what we eat. This is why inflammatory foods have been found to disrupt our health by causing increased symptoms or worsening of symptoms.

I believe that many of us are aware that the food is changing. If you're not familiar with this you must be living under a rock. Most of our vegetables and fruits are grown with hormones, chemicals and pesticides to make them bigger, boost production, delay ripening, make them more colorful and kill mold and insects. Our processed foods are also made with much of the same ingredients including dyes and overly processed oils which are hard for us to digest. While the food industry is thriving off of these changes, the people are getting sick. Many of the chemicals in our foods have already been attributed to conditions such as ADHD, hormone issues, reproductive problems, cancer and immune system issues. Yes, you saw that right, immune system issues. From this we can hypothesize that having any kind of food sitting in your gut for long periods of time can cause digestive issues and be detrimental to your health.

Eating foods that contain good fats, no chemicals or preservatives can be beneficial to improving our gut health. Also adding a fiber supplement or fiber filled foods can improve digestion. Probiotics are an option too to help increase the diverse bacteria in the gut. Taking care of gut issues before they worsen is very important. Many people list digestive issues as a precursor to their MS symptoms and eventually diagnosis. Digestive issues were one of my first symptoms and I should have taken them more seriously. Colon Hydrotherapy or enemas are also options for helping to dissipate gut issues. This involves putting warm water in the rectum through a small tube. Green smoothies and salads can also help produce more bowel movements if constipation is a concern. But taking care of your gut health, making sure waste is constantly moving through the digestive system is a must. Any stagnation can worsen your disease symptoms or produce new ones.

Colon Hydrotherapy

Colon Hydrotherapy aka Colon Cleansing aka Colonics has been around since the Egyptian civilizations. It involves inserting a sterile tube into the rectum and letting purified water slowly go in. This stimulates the colon to perform a motion called peristalsis which causes you to go to the bathroom emptying out feces, mucus, plaque, parasites and more. What does this have to do with MS and other autoimmune diseases? Well if you believe that all disease begins in the gut, why would you not start there for healing? As I discussed previously, many people have digestive issues as a precursor to MS and other disease diagnoses. Numerous doctors have already connected digestive health with physical and mental symptoms that appear in many people. This is why there are so many diets out there for MS. If you are having any kind of nutrient absorption issues, constipation, bloating, gas or any other gastro problems you will need to start with colon hydrotherapy before you start healing. Before I started the Coimbra Protocol (high dose vitamin D) with my functional doctor, she asked me if I had any digestive issues. I found out later that this was to ensure that the nutrients I was putting in would be able to get in my system. Beginning with Colon Hydrotherapy will give you a clean environment to start adding in your new diet and supplements. If you have issues with absorption in the gut because the lining is covered with mucus and plaque, the amount of supplements or healthy foods you eat won't matter. Colon Hydrotherapy is also used in many holistic protocols for Cancer. Regardless of which disease you are trying to heal, a colon cleanse should be first at the top of your to do list.

INFLAMMATION

Inflammation is one of the biggest causes of many diseases today. While inflammation can be good in some situations, we want to prevent the bad inflammation from occurring. Inflammation occurs when the body feels as though it's under attack by a bacteria or virus. It also occurs if there is a part of the body that is hurt or damaged. These are times when inflammation is useful for our bodies. The body activates the immune system and sends inflammatory cells out to address the problem and everything goes back to normal and our bodies are healed. The bad type of inflammation can occur when we are not sick or injured and the body still sends out the same inflammatory cells which end up attacking different parts of our own bodies. No one has figured out why this happens but there are many speculations as to why.

Many people have contributed inflammation to our toxic food supply and certain foods have been proven to make it worse. Inflammation has been linked to saturated fats, stress, dairy products, refined carbohydrates, sugar, sugary drinks, chronic infections, food intolerances and more. Again, this is why diet is extremely important for healing. With MS, we want to make sure that we stay away from products or stressful situations that can cause inflammation in the body and make our symptoms worse. Inflammation can also cause our relapses or flare ups with MS.

SUPPLEMENTS

Supplementation is important for any immune disorder but especially for MS. It has been found that the majority of MS diagnosed people have low vitamin D and trouble absorbing nutrients. This leads us back to the diet and gut health for some! And can you guess what the symptoms of low vitamin D are? You guessed it! Many of the same symptoms of MS and other autoimmune disorders. These include tingling and numbness in the hands and feet, difficulty walking from muscle weakness, muscle and bone pain, twitches and tremors, fatigue, depression and sleep problems. So it is important for us to figure out what your vitamin and nutrient levels are and make sure they are at optimal proportions. This can be done by requesting them from your primary doctor or going to an outpatient blood testing facility. But, this is something that needs to be checked if you are having MS symptoms or have been diagnosed with the disorder. While you may be lacking in other nutrients or vitamins, some of the most common deficiencies for those with MS I listed here.

Magnesium

Magnesium is a common deficiency in most Americans but particularly in those with MS. Magnesium is essential for the body to function and inadequate levels in the body negatively affects the muscles, nerves, blood pressure, heart rate, mood, sleep patterns and more. Many of the symptoms of magnesium deficiency overlap with those of MS and most diagnosed MS people have to take large quantities of this macronutrient. As stated above, a low level of magnesium can affect the nerves, muscles and sleep. MS affects the nerves so anything that can help the nerves keep their myelin sheath and rebuild, us MSer's need. Many People with MS also experience weak muscles and sleep disturbances varying from fatigue to inability to sleep. Magnesium can benefit with this by helping to prevent muscle spasms and relax the body. Many people with MS also struggle with constipation so taking a magnesium supplement can help this as well. Make sure to talk with your doctor to determine your magnesium levels and how it could best benefit you.

Vitamin D3

Vitamin D has been popularized lately by the social media community. More people are finding out about this amazing vitamin which many have recently been calling a hormone. Like magnesium, a deficiency in Vitamin d overlaps with MS symptoms. Tingling feelings, muscle and bone pain, tooth decay, muscle weakness with an inability to walk and more. Are you experiencing any of these Symptoms? We usually get our Vitamin D from sunlight, fish liver oils, salmon, tuna and dairy products. But due to the quality of our current foods we are not getting enough supplementation from them. Also, most people are not outside enough to get the amount of Vitamin D needed from the sun. Not only do you have to be outside but, you would need to have most of your skin exposed to get the proper amount of sunlight needed to produce the body's need of Vitamin D in the body. For darker skinned people, this becomes even more difficult because their skin is a protectant from sunlight. So they would need to be in the sun even longer than a paler person. Let's also add that clouds and smog cover the sun so you're not getting the direct sun rays. No wonder there is a Vitamin D deficiency in America and countries further from the equator. Vitamin D deficiency is already known in the medical world to cause autoimmune disorders such as Type 1 Diabetes, Multiple Sclerosis, Arthritis, Heart Disease, Stroke, Dementia and many Cancers. But most medical doctors are not educated on these new findings and continue to ignore this research. Now that you know this information what will you do with it? If your issue is a Vitamin D deficiency, you want to catch it before it gets worse. Once it gets worse symptoms and disability can become irreversible.

B Complex

B Vitamins are very important to the body and put together they make up the B complex. The B Complex includes B1 (Thiamin), B2 (Riboflavin), B3 (Niacin), B5 (Pantothenic Acid), B6 (Pyridoxine), B9 (Folic Acid) and B12 (Cobalamin). It makes no sense to talk about these separately because they are more potent when taken together. It is necessary to look at your B levels with MS because the B vitamins work together to have a beneficial effect on the nervous system, muscles and heart functions. All issues that MS people have. B Complex can become depleted in the body under extreme stress. Stress is a major precursor to many peoples MS symptoms. If you don't eat much red meat or dairy you could end up with a B vitamin deficiency. If you listen to many people's MS stories, you'll learn that many people were vegan before getting MS. Being vegan is fine if that's what you wish but, you really have to focus on your nutrition as well. Many become deficient in needed nutrients from eating this way.

Multivitamin

At this point everyone should be taking a multivitamin. Children all the way to the elderly. The food is not the same as we discussed earlier. Due to increasing food demands, food is grown faster using chemicals and additives. Important nutrients are left out. A multivitamin just ensures that your levels will not be at zero for certain nutrients and vitamins. All multivitamins are not made equally as well so be careful with which ones you buy. Vitamins are not regulated so many are full of fillers and not so much of the actual nutrients. Read reviews and never go too cheap, especially on something where your health depends on it. Use reputable brands and make sure that the daily value on the label of each nutrient or vitamin is at the minimum of 100%. The brand of the vitamin you choose could be the difference between you putting your autoimmune disorder in remission or not.

Omega 3 Fatty Acids

Omega 3 Fatty Acids are remarkable for us with MS because they can contribute to the rebuilding of the fatty myelin sheath that is getting attacked around the nerves. The myelin sheath is made up of protein and fatty substances and allows electrical impulses to transmit from the brain along the nerve cells to body parts. When the body starts to attack itself, it attacks this myelin sheath interrupting the impulses and leaves actions not completed which shows itself as disability. Some people think the body attacks itself because of the saturated oils. They feel the saturated oils mimic building blocks in our bodies and our immune system gets them confused and tries to attack itself. So we want to stay away from bad fats and the saturated fats found in canola oil, soybean oil, vegetable oil and corn oil. Depending on who you listen to, coconut oil can be either a good oil or bad oil. But the best thing to do is to find out what works for you. It's important to have a diet with good, unsaturated fats in it for MS so that the body has the building blocks to help rebuild the myelin sheath. We want to eat lots of fatty fishes such as salmon, sardines and anchovies. Some people prefer to get their fatty oil in a liquid form. This you can do by taking fish oil, cod liver oil or krill oil. Flaxseeds, walnut oil, hemp oil and many seeds have Omega 3s in them as well. The OMS diet recommends at least 2 tablespoons of flaxseed oil daily and considers it a contributing factor to lessening MS progression. Omega 3's also help to reduce inflammation in the body which is one contributing factor to all autoimmune diseases. They also have been seen to help reduce the risk of breast cancers, cardiovascular diseases, Rheumatoid Arthritis, Alzheimers, blood clots and more.

EXERCISE

Most people hate to hear how they need daily exercise. But, for those of us with an autoimmune disease exercise is extremely important. Have you ever heard of the term "Use it or Lose it"? This is the best term to describe our bodies with MS. We must try to move our bodies and allow the nerves to try to work. If we don't, some of us could lose function. When you have disability, depression and more from a MS diagnosis it's hard to get the motivation to try to workout. I'm not suggesting that you go try to run a 5k or even squat 200lbs. Simple movements can help keep our nerves engaged so that our MS doesn't progress. There is a great group on Facebook called The MS Gym, where there are exercises for those with mobility issues and those without. If you need help you can also visit physical therapy or try e-stim. E-Stim devices stimulate the nerves in the muscles to activate. For those that can move, what are you waiting for? The Best Bet protocol suggests working out daily to not lose any function. Using weights is suggested mostly because it can help strengthen the muscles so they don't atrophy from not being used. Many also think that lifting weights can help the neuron to muscle connection as well. Getting in the gym and being consistent can be hard but it's one of the things that we need to do to fight this disease. If you can't get to the gym, start with chair exercises or just lifting the leg or arm up repeatedly. It will be hard but it will get better. When I first started in the gym I would feel very embarrassed and unstable at times. If on the treadmill I would feel like I was going to fall. Using weights, I felt unsteady. But keep going though, with time and all the changes you are making you will start to feel more stable and sure of yourself.

RELAXATION

MS has already been connected to stress by many doctors and us that have been diagnosed. From school, divorces, deaths, childhood traumas and much more, many started to have their MS symptoms after a traumatic event occurred in their lives. It has been studied that at many times of trauma, our brains can go in flight or fight mode. For those with MS it is said this function did not turn off properly and the hormones released that activated the nervous system are still in the body. Fight or Flight mode is a primitive human function which is said to have been used when humans were hunter gatherers. Fight or Flight mode would help our reaction time when we needed to run from a bear or tiger in the jungle. Or even fight one of these animals. It stimulates the entire nervous system and has been known to make one stronger at the time it is needed. If you have heard of stories where people have had to do extraordinary things such as move a car off of their child or save their children from a burning fire these were likely instances when the person's body was going through Fight or Flight.

To counter this we want to try to relax our nervous systems. With MS, our nervous system is sending signals to attack itself. Anyone, anything or any situation that stresses you or aggravates you, you will need to get away from. If it's a bad marriage, a stress filled job, adult kids…you have to separate yourself from it. Many people who have put themselves in remission meditate or do some kind of mind relaxation techniques to calm their minds. As I stated earlier, one of my first symptoms was the eye twitch that lasted for months. My mind always felt like it was going 100 miles per hour. Little did I know that I was activating my nervous system to go into flight or fight mode. I now meditate at least 3 days a week and try to clear my mind and get my nervous system to relax. Relaxation will be important for your physical body as it heals.

COIMBRA PROTOCOL

The Coimbra Protocol is what I attribute the most to putting my MS in remission. The Coimbra Protocol is named after a Brazilian doctor named Dr. Cicero Coimbra. It is believed that Dr. Coimbra began treating people with MS in 2006. He has helped thousands of people all over the world put their MS and other autoimmune disorders in remission. Dr. Coimbra believes that Vitamin D is not a vitamin but a hormone which controls functions in the body. The Coimbra protocol is done under a doctor's supervision. It involves taking an extremely high dose of Vitamin D along with other supplements, following a low calcium diet and drinking a high amount of water. The dose of your Vitamin D fluctuates depending on your PTH (parathyroid hormone) levels. This is checked monthly by your doctor. When I first started the Coimbra Protocol I could barely walk down my stairs without feeling like I was going to fall. I also couldn't feel the texture of different things with my hands. I could also barely hold a pen. After almost a year, I forgot I had MS. I will say it's not an easy ride though. There were days I felt worse and I questioned if I was doing the right thing. I did have the support of other people with MS through the Facebook group. When I wasn't sure about what was going on or the things I was feeling, I could speak to others there and wait for my doctor to get back to me.

It's important to start the Coimbra Protocol as early as possible. The protocol will not give you back what the disease has taken away but it will stop MS from progressing. I still have slight numbness in my hands and my balance is slightly off. I started almost 6 months after diagnosis and about a year after my first symptoms. This protocol does not work for everyone and depending on who you ask is said to have a success rate of anywhere from 80%-95%. But, because everyone's MS is caused by different issues (remember, MS is only the name of a group of symptoms and those symptoms vary from person to person) I could see this protocol not working if your issue doesn't pertain to Vitamin D. But, as with all the holistic remedies, you will need to investigate and see if it will work for you. I will say that I have seen some remarkable recoveries with MS from those on this protocol.

CCSVI

CCSVI stands for chronic cerebral- spinal venous insufficiency which means impaired blood flow from the brain back to the heart[5]. The term was created by Italian researcher Paulo Zamboni to describe the narrowing of veins in the neck[5]. A link between CCSVI and MS was found in 2009 when a small Italian study reported that 90% of people with MS also had CCSVI[6]. To combat CCSVI a surgery called venoplasty (AKA angioplasty or liberation therapy) is done to open blocked or narrowed veins[6]. While many scientists, doctors and researchers say there is no connection between CCSVI and MS, there have been patients that have had the surgery to un-narrow the veins and have seen benefits. Some have even had all their MS symptoms go away. Still others say that they received limited benefits from the surgery or that their symptoms went away and came back. This could be due to the fact that many say after the veins are widened, they go back to being narrowed after some time. If your blood flow is impaired, a natural way to increase your circulation is exercise. Exercise gets the heart pumping and circulates blood through the body faster.

LDN

LDN, also known as Low Dose naltrexone is an old medication that has more recently been used as an off label drug for autoimmune disorders, cancers, chronic infections and fatigue, pain, inflammation and more. Because LDN is so cheap and cannot be patented or profited from by the pharmaceutical companies, they will not spend money to research it or publicize it. Originally, Naltrexone, was approved for opioid addicts as a way to reduce their pain and addiction when coming off of the drugs[z]. The doses given to addicts were high and were doses of 50mg-100mg[z]. This is completely opposite from the doses that are given for autoimmune disorders. The doses given for autoimmune disorders such as MS are anywhere from 0.001-6mg hence the addition to the name of "Low Dose". The amount of time it takes to feel the effects of Low Dose Naltrexone varies from person to person. Some people, like myself, felt the effects almost immediately. There are others though, where it took up to a year. Most people who the drug works for feel the benefits within a week. I definitely feel like Low Dose Naltrexone helped me get my life back. Another thing is that Low Dose Naltrexone can only be prescribed by a doctor. The issue with this is that most primary doctors are not familiar with the drug. The first time I got my prescription ordered, I had to tell my physician about it and show her information. You may have better luck getting a LDN prescription ordered with a functional doctor or a naturopath.

HSCT

HSCT stands for Hematopoietic Stem Cell Transplant. HSCT is a treatment for MS that has been proven to halt disease progression in many. The goal of HSCT is to reset the immune system and stop inflammation that contributes to MS[1]. HSCT is a serious surgical procedure and its duration is around several months and can take up to a year to recover from. The process of HSCT involves several steps as well. The first step is to start a drug treatment to move stem cells from the bone marrow to the blood for removal[6]. Around 10 days later after this process has been started, the stem cells are removed from the blood and saved for later[6]. Next a chemotherapy infusion is given that wipes out the entire immune system[6]. This process takes several days and requires the patient to be housed in an extreme sanitary and germ free environment since they have no disease protection from their immune system. Later the stem cells are slowly returned to the blood to regrow a new immune system that will not attack itself[6]. The patient continues isolation while the immune system is rebuilding for at least a month.

HSCT is not a treatment to be taken likely and while it has a high completion rate there have been deaths. Also everyone that has completed treatment has not gotten better. There are many people who have stopped their disease progression and regained mobility but still few others who have gotten worse. Currently, HSCT is not FDA approved in the US and is not available unless it's in clinical trials. Many people in the US have had to travel to Mexico, Russia or India to get this treatment and pay out of pocket as they dont take US insurance in those countries. HSCT can get quite expensive as well, ranging anywhere from $30,000- 100,000. Those in the UK have an easier time getting HSCT as a treatment for MS. While there are certain disease requirements, the NHS (National Health Service) and many clinical trials make the treatment available to those with MS and cover the expenses for patients.

SOURCES

1. National MS Society

https://www.nationalmssociety.org/

2. UNM Health Sciences Newsroom

https://hsc.unm.edu/news/2022/02/doctor-researches-toxic-side-effects-rare-earth-metals-mri.html#:~:text=Gadolinium%20is%20a%20rare%20earth,through%20the%20kidneys%20and%20eliminated.

3. Mayo Clinic

https://www.mayoclinic.org/diseases-conditions/multiple-sclerosis/symptoms-causes/syc-20350269#:~:text=Multiple%20sclerosis%20(MS)%20is%20a,the%20rest%20of%20your%20body.

4. Multiple Sclerosis Association of America

https://mymsaa.org/ms-information/overview/types/

5. MS Hope

https://mshope.com/

6. MS Society UK

https://www.mssociety.org.uk/research/explore-
our-research/emerging-research-and-
treatments/chronic-cerebrospinal-venous-
insufficiency---ccsvi

7. LDN Research Trust

https://ldnresearchtrust.org/